Basic Low-Carb Ketogenic Bread Cookbook

50 delicious low-carb recipes for your ketogenic bread, easy to prepare and healthy

I0134874

Raul Wyatt

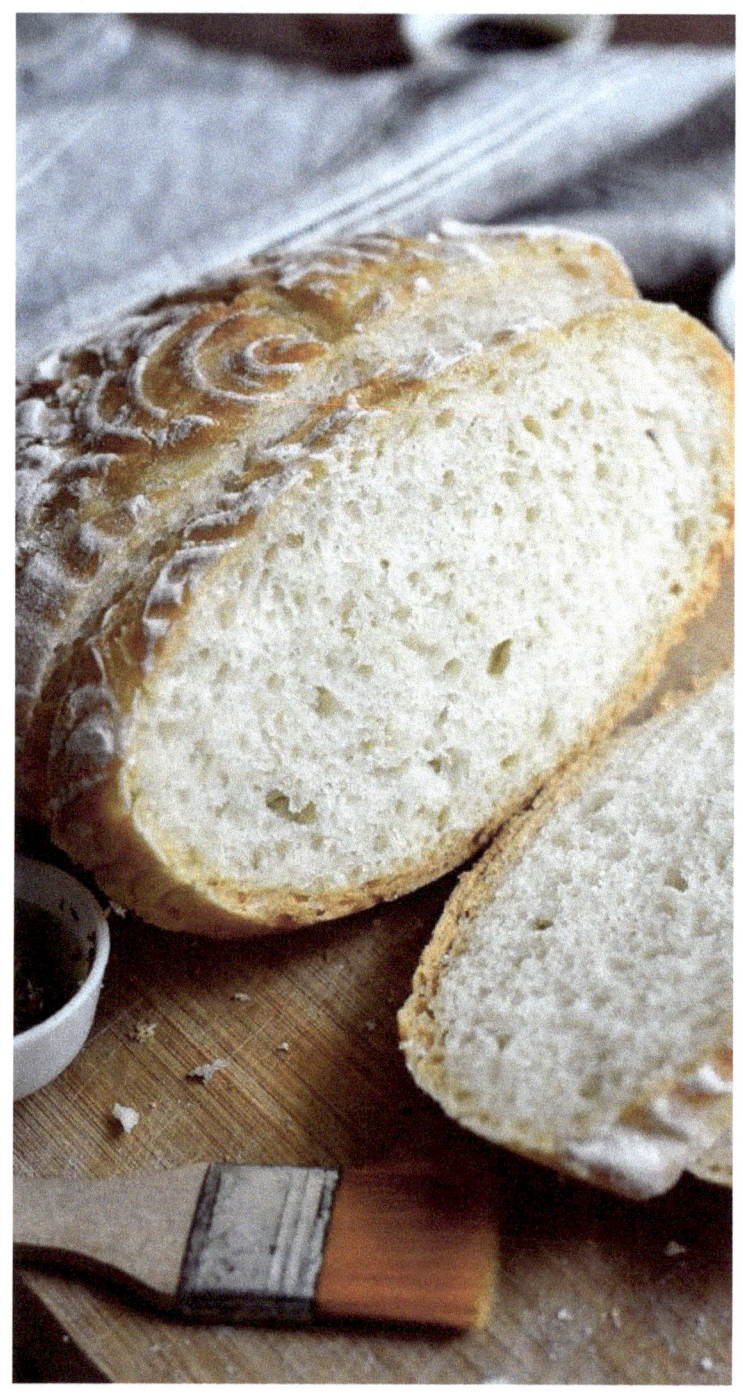

COPYRIGHT

Table of contents

Toast Bread

Preparation time: 3 ½ hours

Cooking time: 3 ½ hours

Servings: 8

Ingredients:

· 1 ½ teaspoons yeast

· 3 cups almond flour

· 2 tablespoons sugar

· 1 teaspoon salt

· 1 ½ tablespoons butter

· 1 cup water

Directions:

1.Pour water into the bowl; add salt, sugar, soft butter, flour, and yeast.

2.I add dried tomatoes and paprika.

3.Put it on the Basic program.

4.The crust can be Light or medium.

Nutrition:

· Carbohydrates: 5 g

· Fats: 2.7 g

· Protein 5.2 g

· Calories: 203

· Fiber: 1 g

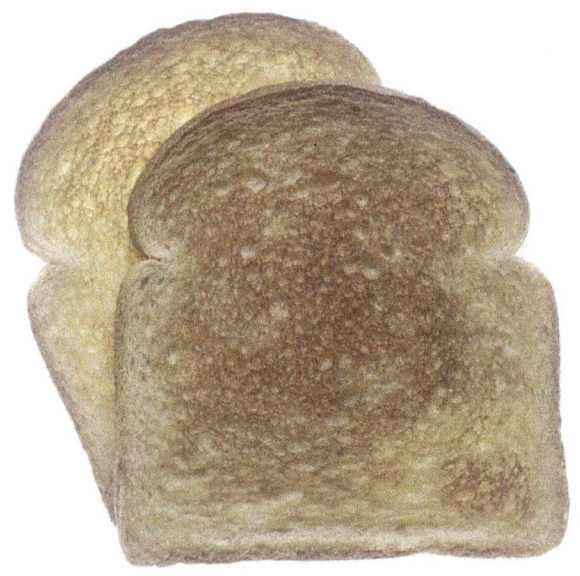

Honey Whole-Wheat Bread

Preparation time: 10 minutes or less

Cooking time: 30 minutes

Ingredients:

8 slices / 1 pound

· ¾ cup water, at 80°F to 90°F

· 1 tablespoon honey

· 1 tablespoon melted butter, cooled

· ½ teaspoon salt

· 2 cups whole-wheat flour

· ½ cup white bread flour

· 1 teaspoon bread machine or instant yeast

12 slices / 1½ pounds

· 1 1/8 cups water, at 80°F to 90°F

· 2 tablespoons honey

· 1½ tablespoons melted butter, cooled

· ¾ teaspoon salt

· 2½ cups whole-wheat flour

· ¾ cup white bread flour

- 1½ teaspoons bread machine or instant yeast

16 slices / 2 pounds

- 1½ cups water, at 80°F to 90°F

- 3 tablespoons honey

- 2 tablespoons melted butter, cooled

- 1 teaspoon salt

- 3¼ cups whole-wheat flour

- 1 cup white bread flour

- 2 teaspoons bread machine or instant yeast

Directions:

1.Place the ingredients in your bread machine as recommended by the manufacturer.

2.Program the machine for Basic/White bread, select Light or medium crust, and press Start.

3.When the loaf is done, remove the bucket from the machine.

4.Let the loaf cool for 5 minutes.

5.Gently shake the bucket to remove the loaf, and turn it out onto a rack to cool.

Ingredient tip: The taste of honey changes depending on what flowers provide the nectar collected by the bees. Try different types of honey, such as robust buckwheat honey or flowery, pale alfalfa honey, to see how the taste of the bread is affected.

Nutrition:

· Calories: 148

· Total fat: 2 g

· Saturated fat: 1 g

· Carbohydrates: 29 g

· Fiber: 1 g

· Protein: 4 g

Crusty French bread

Preparation time: 10 minutes or less

Cooking time: 45 minutes

Ingredients:

8 slices / 1 pound

· 2/3 cup water, at 80°F to 90°F

· 2 teaspoons olive oil

· 1 tablespoon sugar

· 2/3 teaspoon salt

· 2 cups white bread flour

· 1 teaspoon bread machine or instant yeast

12 slices / 1½ pounds

· 1 cup water, at 80°F to 90°F

· 1¼ tablespoons olive oil

· 2 tablespoons sugar

· 1¼ teaspoons salt

· 3 cups white bread flour

· 1¼ teaspoons bread machine or instant yeast

16 slices / 2 pounds

- 1¼ cups water, at 80°F to 90°F

- 1½ tablespoons olive oil

- 2 tablespoons sugar

- 1½ teaspoons salt

- 4 cups white bread flour

- 1½ teaspoons bread machine or instant yeast

Directions:

1.Place the ingredients in your bread machine as recommended by the manufacturer.

2.Program the machine for French bread, select Light or medium crust, and press Start.

3.When the loaf is done, remove the bucket from the machine.

4.Let the loaf cool for 5 minutes.

5.Gently shake the bucket to remove the loaf, and turn it out onto a rack to cool.

Machine tip: If you do not have a French bread setting on your bread machine, use the Basic/White setting and select Medium crust.

Nutrition:

- Calories: 135

- Total fat: 2 g

Bulgur Bread

Preparation time: 3 hours

Cooking time: 3 hours

Servings: 8

Ingredients:

· ½ cup bulgur

· 1/3 cup boiling water

· 1 egg

· 1 cup water

· 1 tablespoon butter

· 1 ½ tablespoon milk powder

· 1 tablespoon sugar

· 2 teaspoons salt

· 3 ¼ cups flour

· 1 teaspoon dried yeast

Directions:

1.Pour bulgur in boiling water into a small container and cover with a lid. Leave to stand for 30 minutes.

2.Cut butter into small cubes.

3.Stir the egg with water in a measuring container. The total volume of eggs with water should be 300 ml.

4.Put all the ingredients in the bread maker in the order that is described in the instructions for your bread maker. Bake in the Basic mode, Medium crust.

Nutrition:

· Carbohydrates: 3 g

· Fat: 3 g

· Protein 8.9 g

· Calories: 255

· Fiber: 1.2 g

100 Percent Whole-Wheat Bread

Preparation time: 10 minutes or less

Cooking time: 45 minutes

Ingredients:

8 slices / 1 pound

· ¾ cup water, at 80°F to 90°F

· 1½ tablespoons melted butter, cooled

· 1½ tablespoons honey

· ¾ teaspoon salt

· 2 cups whole-wheat bread flour

· 1 teaspoon bread machine or instant yeast

12 slices / 1½ pounds

· 1 1/8 cups water, at 80°F to 90°F

· 2¼ tablespoons melted butter, cooled

· 2¼ tablespoons honey

· 1 1/8 teaspoons salt

· 3 cups whole-wheat bread flour

· 1½ teaspoons bread machine or instant yeast

16 slices / 2 pounds

· 1½ cups water, at 80°F to 90°F

· 3 tablespoons melted butter, cooled

· 3 tablespoons honey

· 1½ teaspoons salt

· 3¾ cups whole-wheat bread flour

· 2 teaspoons bread machine or instant yeast

Directions:

1.Place the ingredients in your bread machine as recommended by the manufacturer.

2.Program the machine for Whole-Wheat/Whole-Grain bread, select Light or medium crust, and press Start.

3.When the loaf is done, remove the bucket from the machine.

4.Let the loaf cool for 5 minutes.

5.Gently shake the bucket to remove the loaf, and turn it out onto a rack to cool.

"Did You Know?" Whole-wheat flour contains the entire wheat berry—endosperm, bran, and germ—unlike white flour, which is made up of only the endosperm. This means whole-wheat flour is extremely nutritious and packed with healthy fiber, vitamins, and minerals.

Nutrition:

· Calories: 146

· Total fat: 3 g

· Saturated fat: 1g

· Carbohydrates: 27 g

· Fiber: 1 g

· Protein: 3 g

Walnut Bread

Preparation time: 4 hours

Cooking time: 4 hours

Servings: 10

Ingredients:

· 4 cups almond flour

· ½ cup water

· ½ cup milk

· 2 eggs

· ½ cup walnuts

· 1 tablespoon vegetable oil

· 1 tablespoon sugar

· 1 teaspoon salt

· 1 teaspoon yeast

Directions:

1.All products must be at room temperature.

2.Pour water, milk, and vegetable oil into the bucket and add in the eggs.

3.Now pour in the sifted almond flour. In the process of kneading bread, you may need a little more or less flour — it depends on its moisture.

4.Pour in salt, sugar, and yeast. If it is hot in the kitchen (especially in summer), pour all three ingredients into the different ends of the bucket so that the dough does not have time for peroxide.

5.Now the first kneading dough begins, which lasts 15 minutes. In the process, we monitor the state of the ball. It should be soft, but at the same time, keep its shape and not spread. If the ball does not want to be collected, add a little flour, since the moisture of this product is different for everyone. If the bucket is clean and all the flour is incorporated into the dough, then everything is done right. If the dough is still lumpy and even crumbles, you need to add a little more liquid.

6.Close the lid and then prepare the nuts. They need to be sorted and lightly fried in a dry frying pan; the pieces of nuts will be crispy. Then let them cool and cut with a knife to the desired size. When the bread maker signals, pour in the nuts and wait until the spatula mixes them into the dough.

7.Remove the bucket and take out the walnut bread. Completely cool it on a grill so that the bottom does not get wet.

Nutrition:

· Carbohydrates: 4 g

· Fat: 6.7 g

· Protein: 8.3 g

Everyday White Bread

Preparation time: 10 minutes or less

Cooking time: 20 minutes

Ingredients:

8 slices / 1 pound

· ¾ cup water, at 80°F to 90°F

· 1 tablespoon melted butter, cooled

· 1 tablespoon sugar

· ¾ teaspoon salt

· 2 tablespoons skim milk powder

· 2 cups white bread flour

· ¾ teaspoon bread machine or instant yeast

12 slices / 1½ pounds

· 1 1/8 cups water, at 80°F to 90°F

· 1½ tablespoons melted butter, cooled

· 1½ tablespoons sugar

· 1 teaspoon salt

· 3 tablespoons skim milk powder

· 3 cups white bread flour

· 1¼ teaspoons bread machine or instant yeast

16 slices / 2 pounds

· 1½ cups water, at 80°F to 90°F

· 2 tablespoons melted butter, cooled

· 2 tablespoons sugar

· 2 teaspoons salt

· ¼ cup skim milk powder

· 4 cups white bread flour

· 1½ teaspoons bread machine or instant yeast

Directions:

1.Place the ingredients in your bread machine as recommended by the manufacturer.

2.Program the machine for Basic/White bread, select light or medium crust, and press Start.

3.When the loaf is done, remove the bucket from the machine.

4.Let the loaf cool for 5 minutes.

5.Gently shake the bucket to remove the loaf, and turn it out onto a rack to cool.

"Did You Know?" Powdered milk is usually made from skim milk. This is because the fat particles in regular milk could go rancid, shortening the shelf life of powdered milk, despite the fact that all the water has been removed. Whenever possible, smell the powdered milk, and if there is any odor at all, do not buy it.

Nutrition:

· Calories: 140

· Total fat: 2 g

· Saturated fat: 1 g

· Carbohydrates: 27 g

· Fiber: 1 g

· Protein: 4 g

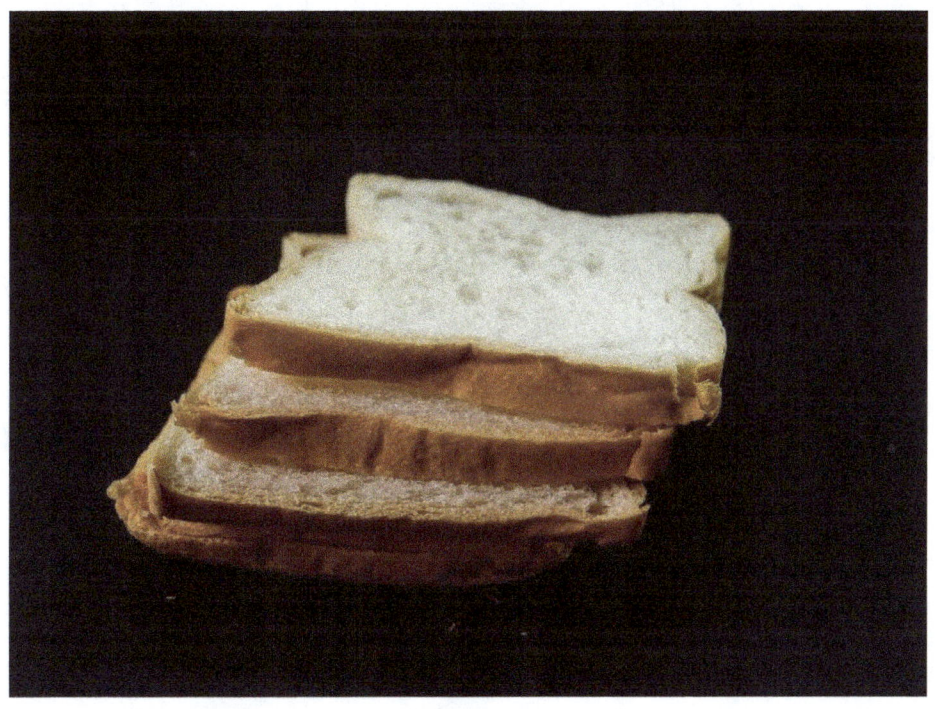

Lovely Oatmeal Bread

Preparation time: 10 minutes or less

Cooking time: 50 minutes

Ingredients:

8 slices / 1 pound

· ¾ cup water, at 80°F to 90°F

· 2 tablespoons melted butter, cooled

· 2 tablespoons sugar

· 1 teaspoon salt

· ¾ cup quick oats

· 1½ cups white bread flour

· 1 teaspoon bread machine or instant yeast

12 slices / 1½ pounds

· 1 1/8 cups water, at 80°F to 90°F

· 3 tablespoons melted butter, cooled

· 3 tablespoons sugar

· 1½ teaspoons salt

· 1 cup quick oats

· 2¼ cups white bread flour

· 1½ teaspoons bread machine or instant yeast

16 slices / 2 pounds

· 1½ cups water, at 80°F to 90°F

· ¼ cup melted butter, cooled

· ¼ cup sugar

· 2 teaspoons salt

· 1½ cups quick oats

· 3 cups white bread flour

· 2 teaspoons bread machine or instant yeast

Directions:

1.Place the ingredients in your bread machine as recommended by the manufacturer.

2.Program the machine for Basic/White bread, select light or medium crust, and press Start.

3.When the loaf is done, remove the bucket from the machine.

4.Let the loaf cool for 5 minutes.

5.Gently shake the bucket to remove the loaf, and turn it out onto a rack to cool.

Ingredient tip: Do not substitute large flake oats for the quick oats in this recipe or the texture will be wrong in your finished bread. Quick oats are chopped up so they absorb liquids easier and cook faster.

Nutrition:

· Calories: 149

· Total fat: 4 g

· Saturated fat: 2 g

· Carbohydrates: 26 g

· Protein: 4 g

Almond Meal Bread

Preparation time: 10 minutes

Cooking time: 4 hours

Servings : 1 ½ pounds / 10 slices

Ingredients:

· 4 eggs, pasteurized

· ¼ cup / 60 ml melted coconut oil

· 1 tablespoon apple cider vinegar

· 2 ¼ cups / 215 grams almond meal

· 1 teaspoon baking soda

· ¼ cup / 35 grams ground flaxseed meal

· 1 teaspoon onion powder

· 1 tablespoon minced garlic

· 1 teaspoon of sea salt

· 1 teaspoon chopped sage leaves

· 1 teaspoon fresh thyme

· 1 teaspoon chopped rosemary leaves

Directions:

1.Gather all the ingredients for the bread and plug in the bread machine having the capacity of 2 pounds of bread recipe.

2.Take a large bowl, crack eggs in it and then beat in coconut oil and vinegar until well blended.

3.Take a separate large bowl, place the almond meal in it, add remaining ingredients, and stir until well mixed.

4.Add egg mixture into the bread bucket, top with flour mixture, shut the lid, select the "basic/white" cycle or "low-carb" setting and then press the Up/down arrow button to adjust baking time according to your bread machine; it will take 3 to 4 hours.

5.Then press the Crust button to select Light crust if available, and press the "start/stop" button to switch on the bread machine.

6.When the bread machine beeps, open the lid, then take out the bread basket and lift out the bread.

7.Let bread cool on a wire rack for 1 hour, then cut it into ten slices and serve.

Nutrition:

· Calories: 104

· Fat: 8.8 g

· Protein: 4 g

· Carbohydrates: 2.1 g

· Fiber: 1.8 g

Pumpernickel Bread

Preparation time: 10 minutes or less

Cooking time: 35 minutes

Ingredients:

8 slices / 1 pound

· ½ cup water, at 80°F to 90°F

· ¼ cup brewed coffee, at 80°F to 90°F

· 2 tablespoons dark molasses

· 5 teaspoons sugar

· 4 teaspoons melted butter, cooled

· 1 tablespoon powdered skim milk

· 1 teaspoon salt

· 4 teaspoons unsweetened cocoa powder

· 2/3 cup dark rye flour

· ½ cup whole-wheat bread flour

· 1 teaspoon caraway seeds

· 1 cup white bread flour

· 1½ teaspoons bread machine or active dry yeast

12 slices / 1½ pounds

· ¾ cup water, at 80°F to 90°F

· 1/3 cup brewed coffee, at 80°F to 90°F

· 3 tablespoons dark molasses

· 2½ tablespoons sugar

· 2 tablespoons melted butter, cooled

· 1½ tablespoons powdered skim milk

· 1½ teaspoons salt

· 2 tablespoons unsweetened cocoa powder

· 1 cup dark rye flour

· ¾ cup whole-wheat bread flour

· 2 teaspoons caraway seeds

· 1½ cups white bread flour

· 2¼ teaspoons bread machine or active dry yeast

16 slices / 2 pounds

· 1 cup water, at 80°F to 90°F

· ½ cup brewed coffee, at 80°F to 90°F

· ¼ cup dark molasses

· 2 tablespoons sugar

· 4 teaspoons melted butter, cooled

· 1 tablespoon powdered skim milk

· 1 teaspoon salt

· 2 tablespoons unsweetened cocoa powder

· 1 1/3 cups dark rye flour

· 1 cup whole-wheat bread flour

· 1 tablespoon caraway seeds

· 2 cups white bread flour

· 2¼ teaspoons bread machine or active dry yeast

Directions:

1.Place the ingredients in your bread machine as recommended by the manufacturer.

2.Program the machine for Basic/White bread, select light or medium crust, and press Start.

3.When the loaf is done, remove the bucket from the machine.

4 .Let the loaf cool for 5 minutes.

5.Gently shake the bucket to remove the loaf, and turn it out onto a rack to cool.

Cooking tip: Rye flour has a very low gluten count, so it does not create fluffy, high-rising loaves of bread. The dough created for rye bread tends to look stickier than other dough, but resist the impulse to add more flour because this will create a tough loaf.

Nutrition:

· Calories: 168

· Total fat: 3 g

· Carbohydrates: 33 g

· Fiber: 4 g

· Protein: 5 g

Sourdough Keto Baguettes

Preparation time: 5 minutes

Cooking time: 17 min

Servings: 10

Dry Ingredients:

· 1/2 cup almond flour (150 g/5.3 oz.)

· 1/3 cup phylum husk powder (40 g/1.4 oz.)

· 1/2 cup coconut flour (60 g/2.1 oz.)

· 1/2 stuffed cup flax supper (75 g/2.6 oz.)

· 1 teaspoon preparing pop

· 1 teaspoon salt (pink Himalayan or ocean salt)

Wet Ingredients:

· 6 large egg whites

· 2 large eggs

· 3/4 cup low-fat buttermilk (180 g/6.5 oz.) — full-fat would make them excessively overwhelming and they may not rise

· 1/4 cup white wine vinegar or apple juice vinegar (60 ml/2 fl oz.)

· 1 cup tepid water (240 ml/8 fl oz.)

Directions:

1.Preheat the broiler to 180 °C/360 °F (fan helped). Use a kitchen scale to gauge every one of the ingredients cautiously. Blend all the dry ingredients in a bowl (almond flour, coconut flour, ground flaxseed, psyllium powder, heating pop, and salt).

2.In a different bowl, blend the eggs, egg whites, and buttermilk.

3.The explanation you shouldn't use just entire eggs is that the bread wouldn't rise with such a large number of egg yolks in. Try not to squander them —use them for making Homemade Mayo, Easy Hollandaise Sauce, or Lemon Curd. For a similar explanation, use low-fat (not full-fat) buttermilk.

4.Add the egg blend and mix them well, using a blender until the mixture is thick. Add vinegar and tepid water and follow procedure until well combined.

5.Don't over-process the mixture. Using a spoon, make 8 ordinary or 16 smaller than usual rolls and place them on a preparing plate fixed with material paper or a non-stick tangle. They will rise, so make a point to leave some space between them. Alternatively, score the loaves slantingly and make 3-4 cuts.

6.Place in the stove and cook for 10 minutes. Then, decrease the temperature to 150 °C/300 °F and heat for another 30-45 minutes (little loaves will set aside because they need less effort to cook).

7.Remove from the stove, let the plate chill off and place the rolls on a rack to chill off to room temperature. Store them at room temperature on the off chance that you intend to use them in the following couple of days or store in the cooler for as long as 3 months.

8 .Cooked products that use psyllium consistently result in a marginally wet surface. If necessary, cut the rolls down the middle and place in a toaster or in the broiler before serving.

Tip: To spare time, blend all the dry ingredients ahead and store in a zip-lock sack, and add a mark with the number of servings. At the point when fit to be prepared, simply include the wet ingredients!

Nutrition:

· Calories: 21

· Fat: 4.7 g

· Carbohydrates: 44.2 g

· Protein: 0 g

· Sugars: 5 g

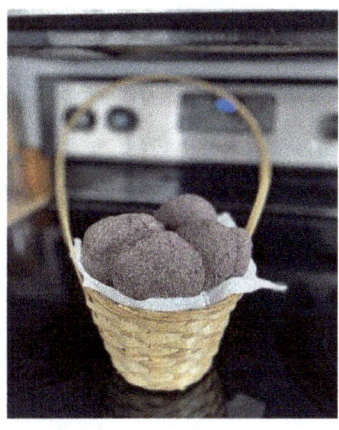

Zucchini Bread for keto diet

Preparation time: 15 minutes

Cooking time: 58 min

Servings: 12

Ingredients:

· 3 ounces almond flour

· 2 ounces coconut flour

· 1/2 teaspoon salt

· 1/2 teaspoon pepper

· 2 teaspoons heating powder

· 1 teaspoon thickener

· 5 large eggs

· 2/3 cup margarine, melted

· 4 ounces Cheddar, ground

· 6 ounces zucchini, ground, and fluid crushed out

· 6 ounces bacon, diced

Directions:

1.Preheat broiler to 175°C/350°F.

2.In a big bowl, add the almond flour, coconut flour, salt, pepper, preparing powder, and thickener. Blend well.

3.Add the eggs and softened spread and blend well.

4.Overlap through ¾ of the Cheddar, alongside the zucchini and bacon.

5.Spoon into your moisture 9-inches clay portion dish (if using a meat dish, line with material paper) and cook for 35 minutes, remove from the stove, and top with the rest of the Cheddar.

6.Cook for another 10-15 minutes, until the cheddar has caramelized and a stick comes out clean.

7.Leave to cool for 20 minutes.

8.Cut into 12 cuts and enjoy warm.

Nutrition:

· Calories: 270

· Fat: 15 g

· Fiber: 3 g

· Carbohydrates: 5 g

· Protein: 9 g

French Ham Bread

Preparation time: 3 hours 30 minutes

Cooking time: 3 hours 30 minutes

Servings: 8

Ingredients:

· 3 1/3 cups Almond flour

· 1 cup ham

· ½ cup milk powder

· 1 ½ tablespoons sugar

· 1 teaspoon yeast, fresh

· 1 teaspoon salt

· 1 teaspoon dried basil

· 1 1/3 cups water

· 2 tablespoons olive oil

Directions:

1.Cut ham into cubes of 0.5-1 cm (approximately ¼ inch).

2.Put the ingredients in the bread maker in the following order: water, olive oil, salt, sugar, flour, milk powder, ham, and yeast.

3.Put all the ingredients according to the instructions to your bread maker.

4.Put basil in a dispenser or fill it later at the signal in the container.

5.Turn on the bread machine.

6.After the end of the Baking cycle, leave the bread container in the bread maker to keep warm for 1 hour.

7.Then your delicious bread is ready!

Nutrition:

· Carbohydrates: 2 g

· Fats: 5.5 g

· Protein: 11.4 g

· Calories: 287

· Fiber: 1 g

Molasses Wheat Bread

Preparation time: 10 minutes or less

Cooking time: 1 hour 30 minutes

Ingredients:

8 slices / 1 pound

· ½ cup water, at 80°F to 90°F

· 1/4 cup milk, at 80°F

· 2 teaspoons melted butter, cooled

· 2 tablespoons honey

· 1 tablespoon molasses

· 1 teaspoon sugar

· 1 tablespoon skim milk powder

· ½ teaspoon salt

· 1 teaspoon unsweetened cocoa powder

· 1¼ cups whole-wheat flour

· 1 cup white bread flour

· 1 teaspoon bread machine yeast or instant yeast

12 slices / 1½ pounds

· ¾ cup water, at 80°F to 90°F

- 1/3 cup milk, at 80°F

- 1 tablespoon melted butter, cooled

- 3¾ tablespoons honey

- 2 tablespoons molasses

- 2 teaspoons sugar

- 2 tablespoons skim milk powder

- ¾ teaspoon salt

- 2 teaspoons unsweetened cocoa powder

- 1¾ cups whole-wheat flour

- 1¼ cups white bread flour

- 1 1/8 teaspoons bread machine yeast or instant yeast

16 slices / 2 pounds

- 1 cup water, at 80°F to 90°F

- ½ cup milk, at 80°F

- 2 tablespoons melted butter, cooled

- 5 tablespoons honey

- 3 tablespoons molasses

- 1 tablespoon sugar

- 3 tablespoons skim milk powder

- 1 teaspoon salt

- 1 tablespoon unsweetened cocoa powder

· 2½ cups whole-wheat flour

· 2 cups white bread flour

· 1½ teaspoons bread machine or instant yeast

Directions:

1.Place the ingredients in your bread machine as recommended by the manufacturer.

2.Program the machine for Basic/White bread, select light or medium crust, and press Start.

3.When the loaf is done, remove the bucket from the machine.

4.Let the loaf cool for 5 minutes.

5.Gently shake the bucket to remove the loaf, and turn it out onto a rack to cool.

Ingredient tip: Look for unsulphured molasses because it is sweeter and lacks the slight chemical taste of sulphured products. Also, this bread is best with sticky, rich dark or blackstrap molasses instead of light-colored molasses.

Nutrition:

· Calories: 164

· Total fat: 2 g

· Saturated fat: 1 g

· Carbohydrates: 34 g

Oat Bran Molasses Bread

Preparation time: 10 minutes or less

Cooking time: 40 minutes

Ingredients:

8 slices / 1 pound

· ½ cup water, at 80°F to 90°F

· 1½ tablespoons melted butter, cooled

· 2 tablespoons blackstrap molasses

· ¼ teaspoon salt

· 1/8 teaspoon ground nutmeg

· ½ cup oat bran

· 1½ cups whole-wheat bread flour

· 1 1/8 teaspoons bread machine or instant yeast

12 slices / 1½ pounds

· ¾ cup water, at 80°F to 90°F

· 2¼ tablespoons melted butter, cooled

· 3 tablespoons blackstrap molasses

· 1/3 teaspoon salt

· ¼ teaspoon ground nutmeg

- ¾ cup oat bran

- 2¼ cups whole-wheat bread flour

- 1¾ teaspoons bread machine or instant yeast

16 slices / 2 pounds

- 1 cup water, at 80°F to 90°F

- 3 tablespoons melted butter, cooled

- ¼ cup blackstrap molasses

- ½ teaspoon salt

- ¼ teaspoon ground nutmeg

- 1 cup oat bran

- 3 cups whole-wheat bread flour

- 2¼ teaspoons bread machine or instant yeast

Directions:

1.Place the ingredients in your bread machine as recommended by the manufacturer.

2.Program the machine for Whole-Wheat/Whole-Grain bread, select light or medium crust, and press Start.

3.When the loaf is done, remove the bucket from the machine.

4.Let the loaf cool for 5 minutes.

5.Gently shake the bucket to remove the loaf, and turn it out onto a rack to cool.

Decoration tip: Lightly brush the warm loaf with melted butter when you pop it out of the bucket, and scatter toasted whole oats on the top. The butter will create a lovely, soft crust and allow the oats to stick.

Nutrition:

· Calories: 137

· Total fat: 3 g

· Saturated fat: 2 g

· Carbohydrates: 25 g

· Fiber: 1 g

· Protein: 3 g

Milk Almond Bread

Preparation time: 3 ½ hours

Cooking time: 3 ½ hours

Servings: 8

Ingredients:

· 1 ¼ cup milk

· 5 ¼ cups almond flour

· 2 tablespoons butter

· 2 teaspoons dry yeast

· 1 tablespoon sugar

· 2 teaspoons salt

Directions:

1.Pour the milk into the form and ½ cup of water. Add flour.

2.Put butter, sugar, and salt in different corners of the mold. Make a groove in the flour and put in the yeast.

3.Bake on the Basic program.

4.Cool the bread.

Nutrition:

· Carbohydrates: 5 g

· Fats: 4.5 g

· Protein: 10.1 g

· Calories: 352

· Fiber:: 1,5 g

Bread for keto diet

Preparation time: 15 minutes

Cooking time: 40 min

Servings: 6

Ingredients:

· 2 cups fine ground almond dinner (from whitened almonds)

· 2 teaspoons preparing powder

· 1/2 teaspoon fine Himalayan salt

· 1/2 cup olive oil or avocado oil

· 1/2 cup separated water

· 5 large eggs

· 1 tablespoon poppy seeds

Directions:

1.You will require a hand blender, portion dish, and material paper.

2.Pre-heat stove to 400°F. Line portion container with material paper.

3.In a large bowl, combine the almond dinner, preparing powder and salt.

4.While as yet blending, shower in the avocado oil until a brittle batter structure. Make a well (little gap) in the mixture.

5.Air out the eggs into the well, add the water, and beat together, making little circles with your blender in the eggs until light yellow and foamy. Then, start making greater circles to fuse the almond feast and blend into it. Continue blending like this, until it would appear that flapjack hitter— Smooth, light, and thick.

6.Empty the blend into the portion container, use a spatula to scratch it full scale. Sprinkle the poppy seeds on top. Heat for 40 minutes in the middle rack. It will be hard, raised, and brilliant dark colored when done.

7.Remove from the broiler and let it sit for 30 minutes to cool. Then, unmold and cut it.

8.Store in water/airproof compartment in the ice chest as long as 5 days. Toast to warm!

Nutrition:

· Calories: 270

· Fat: 15 g

· Fiber:: 3 g

· Carbohydrates: 5 g

· Protein: 9 g

Sausage bread

Preparation time: 4 hours

Cooking time: 4 hours

Servings: 8

Ingredients:

· 1 ½ teaspoons dry yeast

· 3 cups flour

· 1 teaspoon sugar

· 1 ½ teaspoons salt

· 1 1/3 cups whey

· 1 tablespoon oil

· 1 cup chopped smoked sausage

Directions:

1.Add all the ingredients in the order that is recommended specifically for your model.

2.Set the required parameters for Baking bread.

3.When ready, remove the delicious hot bread.

4.Wait for it to cool down and enjoy with sausage.

Nutrition:

· Carbohydrates: 4 g

· Fats: 5.1 g

· Protein: 7.4 g

· Calories: 234

· Fiber: 1,3 g

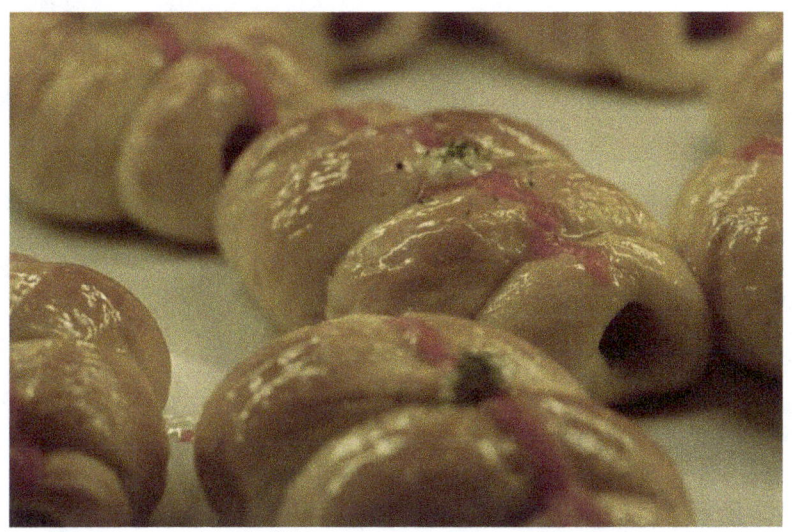

Gluten-Free Chocolate Zucchini Bread

Preparation time: 5 minutes

Cooking time: 10 minutes

Servings: 12

Ingredients:

· 1 ½ cups coconut flour

· ¼ cup unsweetened cocoa powder

· ½ cup erythritol

· ½ teaspoon cinnamon

· 1 teaspoon baking soda

· 1 teaspoon baking powder

· ¼ teaspoon salt

· ¼ cup coconut oil, melted

· 4 eggs

· 1 teaspoon vanilla

· 2 cups zucchini, shredded

Directions:

1.Shred the zucchini and use paper towels to drain excess water, set aside.

2.Lightly beat eggs with coconut oil, then add to bread machine pan.

3.Add the remaining ingredients to the pan.

4.Set bread machine to Gluten-free.

5.When the bread is done, remove the bread machine pan from the bread machine.

6.Let it cool slightly before transferring to a cooling rack.

7.You can store your bread for up to 5 days.

Nutrition:

· Calories: 185

· Carbohydrates: 6 g

· Fats: 17 g

· Protein: 5 g

Zucchini Bread

Preparation time: 2 hours 10 minutes

Cooking time: 2 hours 10 minutes

Servings: 8

Ingredients:

· 2 whole eggs

· ¼ teaspoon sea salt

· 1 cup olive oil

· 1 cup white sugar

· 1 tablespoon vanilla sugar

· 2 teaspoons cinnamon

· ½ cup nuts, ground

· 3 cups bread flour, well sifted

· 1 tablespoon baking powder

· 1¼ cup zucchini, grated

Directions:

1.Prepare all of the ingredients for your bread and measuring utensils (a cup, a spoon, kitchen scales).

2.Carefully measure the ingredients into the pan, except the zucchini and nuts.

3.Place all the ingredients into the bread bucket in the right order, following the manual for your bread machine.

4.Close the cover.

5.Select the program of your bread machine to Cake and choose the crust color to Light.

6.Press Start.

7.After the signal, put the grated zucchini and nuts into the dough.

8.Wait until the program completes.

9.When done, take the bucket out and let it cool for 5-10 minutes.

10. Shake the loaf from the pan and let it cool for 30 minutes on a cooling rack.

11. Slice, serve, and enjoy the taste of fragrant homemade bread.

Nutrition:

· Carbohydrates: 4 g

· Fats: 31 g

· Protein: 8.6 g

· Calories: 556

· Fiber: 1.3 g

Apple Butter Bread

Preparation time: 2 hours

Cooking time: 25 minutes

Servings: 10

Ingredients:

· ½ cup unsalted melted butter

· 1 cup swerve sweetener

· 1 egg

· 1 cup unsweetened apple butter

· 1 teaspoon of cinnamon powder

· 2 cups almond flour

· 2 teaspoons baking soda

· 1 teaspoon nutmeg ground

· 1 teaspoon extract of vanilla

· ½ cup of unsweetened almond milk

· 2 teaspoons of active dry yeast

Directions:

1.Mix the almond flour, Swerve, cinnamon, nutmeg powder, and baking soda in a container.

2.Get another container and combine the unsweetened apple butter, unsalted melted butter, vanilla essence, and almond milk that are unsweetened.

3.As per the instructions on the manual of your machine, pour the ingredients in the bread pan, taking care to follow how to mix in the yeast.

4.Place the bread pan in the machine and select the Sweet bread setting, together with the crust type, if available, then press Start once you have closed the lid of the machine.

5.When the bread is ready, using oven mitts, remove the bread pan from the machine. Use a stainless spatula to extract the bread from the pan and turn the pan upside down on a metallic rack where the bread will cool off before slicing it.

Nutrition:

· Calories: 217

· Fat: 13 g

· Carbohydrates: 42 g

· Protein: 4 g

Egg Coconut Bread

Preparation time: 10 minutes

Cooking time: 40 minutes

Servings: 4

Ingredients:

· ½ cup coconut flour

· 4 eggs

· 1 cup water

· 2 tablespoons apple cider vinegar

· ¼ cup coconut oil, plus 1 teaspoon melted

· ½ teaspoon garlic powder

· ½ teaspoon baking soda

· ¼ teaspoon salt

Directions:

1.Preheat the oven to 350°F.

2.Grease a baking tin with 1 teaspoon coconut oil. Set aside.

3.Add eggs to a blender along with vinegar, water, and ¼-cup coconut oil. Blend for 30 seconds.

4.Add coconut flour, baking soda, garlic powder, and salt. Blend for 1 minute.

5.Transfer to the baking tin.

6.Bake for 40 minutes.

7.Enjoy.

Nutrition:

· Calories: 297

· Fat: 14 g

· Carbohydrates: 9 g

· Protein: 15 g

Coconut Milk Bread

Preparation time: 10 minutes

Cooking time: 3 hours

Servings: 10

Ingredients:

· 1 whole egg

· ½ cup lukewarm milk

· ½ cup lukewarm coconut milk

· ¼ cup butter, melted and cooled

· 2 tablespoons liquid honey

· 4 cups almond flour, sifted

· 1 tablespoon active dry yeast

· 1 teaspoon salt

· ½ cup coconut chips

Directions:

1.Prepare all the ingredients for your bread and measuring utensils (a cup, a spoon, kitchen scales).

2.Carefully measure the ingredients into the pan, except the coconut chips.

3.Place all the ingredients into the bread bucket in the right order, following the manual for your bread machine.

4.Close the cover.

5.Select the program of the bread machine to Sweet and choose the crust color to Medium.

6.Press Start.

7.After the signal, add the coconut chips into the dough.

8.Wait until the program completes.

9.When done, take the bucket out and let it cool for 5-10 minutes.

10. Shake the loaf from the pan and let it cool for 30 minutes on a cooling rack.

11. Slice, serve, and enjoy the taste of fragrant homemade bread.

Nutrition:

· Carbohydrates: 6 g

· Fats: 15.3 g

· Protein: 9.5 g

· Calories: 421

· Fiber: 1.6 g

Cheese Sausage Bread

Preparation time: 4 hours

Cooking time: 4 hours

Servings: 8

Ingredients:

· 1 teaspoon dry yeast

· 3 ½ cups flour

· 1 teaspoon salt

· 1 tablespoon sugar

· 1 ½ tablespoon oil

· 2 tablespoons smoked sausage

· 2 tablespoons grated cheese

· 1 tablespoon chopped garlic

· 1 cup water

Directions:

1.Cut the sausage into small cubes.

2.Grate the cheese on a grater; chop the garlic.

3.Add the ingredients to the bread machine according to the instructions.

4.Turn on the baking program, and let it do the work.

Nutrition:

· Carbohydrates: 4 g

· Fats: 5.6 g

· Protein: 7.7 g

· Calories: 260

· Fiber:: 1.3 g

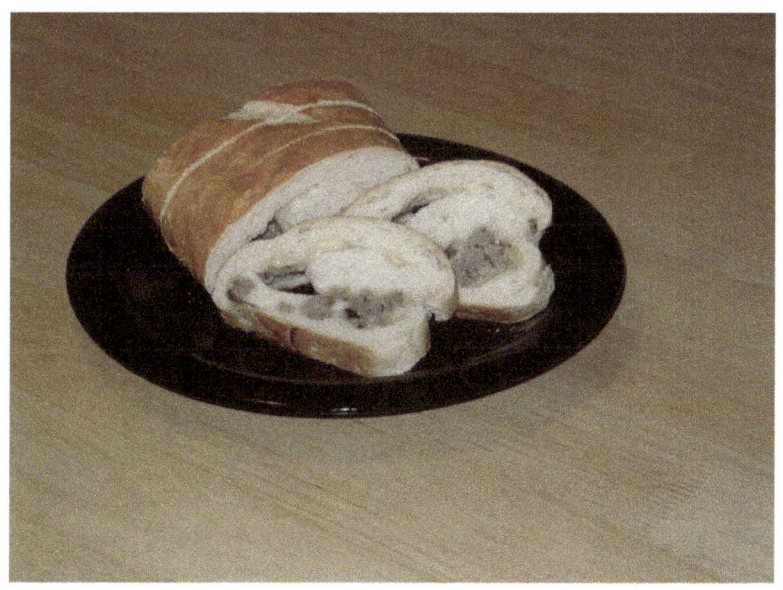

Lemon Blueberry Bread

Preparation time: 2 hours

Cooking time: 25 minutes

Servings: 10

Ingredients:

· 2 cups almond flour

· 1/2 cup coconut flour

· 1/2 cup g hee

· 1/2 cup coconut oil, melted

· 1/2 cup erythritol

· 4 eggs

· 2 tablespoons l emon zest , about half a lemon

· 1 teaspoon l emon juice

· 1/2 cup blueberries

· 2 teaspoons baking powder

Directions:

1.Lightly beat eggs before pouring them into your bread machine pan.

2.Add melted coconut oil, ghee, and lemon juice to the pan.

3.Add the remaining dry ingredients including blueberries and lemon zest to the bread machine pan.

4.Set bread machine to Quick bread setting.

5.When the bread is done, remove the bread machine pan from the bread machine.

6.Let it cool slightly before transferring to a cooling rack.

7.You can store your bread for up to 5 days.

Nutrition:

· Calories: 300

· Carbohydrates: 14 g

· Protein: 5 g

· Fat: 30 g

Sweet Coffee Bread

Preparation time: 2 hours

Cooking time: 25 minutes

Servings: 10

Ingredients:

· 2 cups of almond fine flour

· ½ teaspoon salt

· Cinnamon, three-quarters of a teaspoon

· 4 eggs

· ½ cup Swerve Keto sweetener

· ½ cup of unsalted melted butter

· ¼ cup of protein powder that is not flavored

· 4 teaspoons of coconut flour

· 2/3 cup of almond milk that is not sweetened

· 2 teaspoons espresso

· ½ teaspoon extract from vanilla

· 2 teaspoons active dry yeast

· 2 teaspoons baking powder

Directions:

1.Mix together the almond flour, coconut flour, sweetener Swerve, cinnamon, salt, baking powder, espresso, and unflavored protein powder in a container.

2.Mix the unsweetened almond milk, eggs, extract of vanilla, and unsalted melted butter in another container.

3.As per the instructions on the manual of your machine, pour the ingredients in the bread pan, taking care to follow how to mix in the yeast.

4.Place the bread pan in the machine, and select the Sweet bread setting, together with the crust type, if available, then press Start once you have closed the lid of the machine.

5.When the bread is ready, extract it from the pan and place it on a wire mesh surface to cool before cutting it.

Nutrition:

· Calories: 177

· Fat: 3.8 g

· Carbohydrates: 31 g

· Protein: 4.6 g

Bread with Beef

Preparation time: 2 hours

Cooking time: 2 hours

Servings: 6

Ingredients:

· 5 oz. beef

· 15 oz. almond flour

· 5 oz. rye flour

· 1 onion

· 3 teaspoons dry yeast

· 5 tablespoons olive oil

· 1 tablespoon sugar

· Sea salt

· Ground black pepper

Directions:

1.Pour the warm water into the 15 oz. of the wheat flour and rye flour and leave overnight.

2.Chop the onions and cut the beef into cubes.

3.Fry the onions until clear and golden brown and then mix in the bacon and fry on low heat for 20 minutes until soft.

4.Combine the yeast with the warm water, mixing until smooth consistency, and then combine the yeast with the flour, salt and sugar, but don't forget to mix and knead well.

5.Add in the fried onions with the beef and black pepper and mix well.

6.Pour some oil into a bread machine and place the dough into the bread maker. Cover the dough with the towel and leave for 1 hour.

7.Close the lid and turn the bread machine on the Basic/white bread program.

8.Bake the bread until the medium crust and after the bread is ready take it out and leave for 1 hour covered with the towel and only then you can slice the bread.

Nutrition:

· Carbohydrates: 6 g

· Fats: 21 g

· Protein: 13 g

· Calories: 299

· Fiber: 1.6 g

Cinnamon Cake

Preparation time: 7 minutes

Cooking time: 5 minutes

Servings: 12

Ingredients:

· ½ cup erythritol

· ½ cup butter

· ½ tablespoon vanilla extract

· 1 ¾ cups almond flour

· 1 ½ teaspoons baking powder

· 1 ½ teaspoons cinnamon

· ¼ teaspoon sea salt

· 1 ½ cups carrots, grated

· 1 cup pecans, chopped

Directions:

1.Grate carrots and place them in a food processor.

2.Add in the rest of the ingredients, except the pecans, and process until well incorporated.

3.Fold in pecans.

4.Pour mixture into bread machine pan.

5.Set bread machine to Bake.

6.When baking is completed, remove from the bread machine and transfer to a cooling rack.

7.Allow cooling completely before slicing. (You can also top with a sugar-free cream cheese frosting, see recipe below).

8.You can store it for up to 5 days in the refrigerator.

Nutrition:

· Calories: 350

· Carbohydrates: 8 g

· Fats: 34 g

· Protein: 7 g

Cream Cheese Bread

Preparation time: 10 minutes

Cooking time: 4 hours

Servings: 1 ½ pounds / 12 slices

Ingredients:

· ¼ cup / 60 grams butter, grass-fed, unsalted

· 1 cup and 3 tablespoons / 140 grams cream cheese, softened

· 4 egg yolks, pasteurized

· 1 teaspoon vanilla extract, unsweetened

· 1 teaspoon baking powder

· ¼ teaspoon of sea salt

· 2 tablespoons monk fruit powder

· ½ cup / 65 grams peanut flour

Directions:

1.Gather all the ingredients for the bread and plug in the bread machine having the capacity of 2 pounds of bread recipe.

2.Take a large bowl, place butter in it, beat in cream cheese until thoroughly combined, and then beat in egg yolks, vanilla, baking powder, salt, and monk fruit powder until well combined.

3.Add egg mixture into the bread bucket, top with flour, shut the lid, select the "basic/white" cycle or "low-carb" setting and then press the Up/Down arrow button to adjust baking time according to your bread machine; it will take 3 to 4 hours.

4.Then press the Crust button to select Light crust if available, and press the "start/stop" button to switch on the bread machine.

5.When the bread machine beeps, open the lid, then take out the bread basket and lift out the bread.

6.Let bread cool on a wire rack for 1 hour, then cut it into twelve slices and serve.

Nutrition:

· Calories: 98

· Fat: 7.9 g

· Protein: 3.5 g

· Carbohydrates: 2.6 g

· Fiber: 0.4 g

· Net Carb: 2.2 g

Banana Bread

Preparation time: 2 hours

Cooking time: 30 minutes

Servings: 12

Ingredients:

· 2 cups almond flour

· 1/4 cup coconut flour

· 1/2 cup walnuts, chopped

· 2 teaspoons baking powder

· 2 teaspoons cinnamon

· 1/4 teaspoon Himalayan salt

· 6 tablespoons coconut oil, melted

· 1/2 cup erythritol

· 4 eggs

· 1/4 cup a lmond milk , unsweetened

· 2 teaspoons b anana extract

· 1/2 teaspoon xanthan gum

Directions:

1.Place all the wet ingredients into the pan of the bread machine.

2.Add all dry ingredients next.

3.Set bread machine to Quick bread setting.

4.When the bread is done, remove the bread machine pan from the bread machine.

5.Let it cool slightly before transferring to a cooling rack.

6.You can store your bread for up to 5 days.

Nutrition:

· Calories: 224

· Carbohydrates: 6 g

· Protein: 8 g

· Fat: 20 g

Great Flavor Cheese Bread With the Added Kick of Pimento Olives

Preparation time: 5 minutes

Cooking time: 3 hours

Servings: 1 loaf

Ingredients:

· 1 cup water room temperature

· 4 teaspoons sugar

· 3/4 teaspoon salt

· 1 ¼ cups shredded sharp Cheddar cheese

· 3 cups bread flour

· 2 teaspoons active dry yeast

· 3/4 cup pimiento olives, drained and sliced

Direction:

1.Add all ingredients except olives to the machine pan.

2.Select Basic bread setting.

3.At prompt before second knead, mix in olives.

Nutrition:

· Calories: 124

· Total fat: 4 g (2 g sat. fat),

· Carb. 19 g

· Fiber: 1 g

· Protein: 5 g

Wild Rice Cranberry Bread

Preparation time: 5 minutes

Cooking time: 3 hours

Servings: 1 loaf

Ingredients:

· 1 ¼ cup water

· ¼ cup skim milk powder

· 1 ¼ teaspoon salt

· 2 tablespoons liquid honey

· 1 tablespoon extra-virgin olive oil

· 3 cups all-purpose flour

· 3/4 cup cooked wild rice

· 1/4 cup pine nuts

· ¾ teaspoon celery seeds

· 1/8 teaspoon freshly ground black pepper

· 1 teaspoon bread machine or instant yeast

· 2/3 cup dried cranberries

Direction:

1.Add all ingredients to the machine pan except the cranberries.

2.Place pan into the oven chamber.

3.Select Basic bread setting.

4.At the signal to add ingredients, add the cranberries.

Nutrition:

· Calories: 225

· Total fat: 7.8 g (1.2 g sat. fat)

· Carb: 33 g

· Fiber: 1 g

· Protein: 6,7 g

Fantastic Bread

Preparation time: 5 minutes

Cooking time: 20 min

Servings: 6

Ingredients:

· 1 cup almond flour or almond supper

· 4 tablespoons entire psyllium husk

· 2 teaspoons of preparing powder

· 1/2 teaspoon of salt (discretionary) little bunch almond fragments (discretionary) little bunch squashed pecans

· 6 large eggs

· 1 cup full-fat yogurt

Directions:

1.Add the dry ingredients to a big blending bowl and mix. The nuts are discretionary or can fill in for different kinds of nuts on the off chance that you like.

2.Crack 6 large eggs into a different blending bowl, add one cup of full-fat yogurt, and blend well in with a hand blender. Add the dry blend and blend completely with a hand blender. Set it aside for 10–15 minutes while you preheat your broiler to 350° F.

3.Rinse the material paper under warm water and shake it off before crushing it into your preparing tin, then add your blend to the tin and press it into the sides. You can add nuts like almonds, sesame seeds, and pumpkin seeds to the highest point of the portion and pop it into the stove for 55 minutes. Haul the bread out when completed and let it cool on a rack.

Nutrition:

· Calories: 40

· Carbohydratess: 4 g

· Net Carbohydratess: 2.5 g

· Fiber: 5.5 g

· Fat: 9 g

· Protein: 6 g

· Sugars: 3 g

Cheese Cauliflower Broccoli Bread

Preparation time: 10 minutes

Cooking time: 3 hours

Servings : 1 loaf

Ingredients:

· 1/4 cup water

· 4 tablespoons oil

· 1 egg white

· 1 teaspoon lemon juice

· 2/3 cup grated Cheddar cheese

· 3 tablespoons green onion

· 1/2 cup broccoli, chopped

· 1/2 cup cauliflower, chopped

· 1/2 teaspoon lemon-pepper seasoning

· 2 cup bread flour

· 1 teaspoon regular or quick-rising yeast

Direction:

1.Add all ingredients to the machine pan.

2.Select Basic bread setting.

Nutrition:

· Calories:156

· Total fat: 7.4 g (2.2 g sat. fat)

· Carb:17 g

· Fiber: 0 g

· Protein: 4.9 g

Ricotta Chive Bread

Preparation time: 5 minutes

Cooking time: 3 hours

Servings: 1 loaf

Ingredients:

· 1 cup lukewarm water

· 1/3 cup whole or part-skim ricotta cheese

· 1 ½ teaspoon salt

· 1 tablespoon granulated sugar

· 3 cups bread flour

· 1/2 cup chopped chives

· 2 ½ teaspoon instant yeast

Direction:

1.Add ingredients to bread machine pan except for dried fruit.

2.Choose the Basic bread setting and Light/medium crust.

Nutrition:

· Calories: 92

Keto English Muffin Loaf

Preparation time: 10 minutes

Cooking time: 3 hours

Total Time: 3 hours 10 minutes

Servings: 1-pound loaf of 8 slices

Ingredients:

· 1 cup warm water (80 °F)

· 2 tablespoons Sugar

· 3 tablespoons Non-fat dry milk

· 1 teaspoon salt

· ¼ teaspoon baking soda

· 2 ½ cups almond flour

· 1 tablespoon vital wheat gluten

· 1 ¾ teaspoon dry active yeast

Directions:

1.Measure all the ingredients in the bread machine pan in the order listed above.

2.Turn on the bread machine and process. Select Basic cycle; choose normal Crust Color setting. Close the lid and press the Start button.

3.Once cooked, place bread in a cooling rack.

4.Slice, then toast and serve.

Nutrition:

· Calories: 22

· Calories from fat: 9

· Total Fat: 1 g

· Total Carbohydrates: 3 g

· Net Carbohydrates: 3 g

· Protein: 2g

Celery Bread

Preparation time: 10 minutes

Cooking time: 3 hours

Servings: 1 loaf

Ingredients:

· 1 (10 oz.) can cream of celery soup

· 3 tablespoons low-fat milk, heated

· 1 tablespoon vegetable oil

· 1 ¼ teaspoons celery, garlic, or onion salt

· 3/4 cup celery, fresh/slice thin

· 1 tablespoon celery leaves, fresh, chopped -optional

· 1 egg

· 3 cups bread flour

· 1/4 teaspoon sugar

· 1/4 teaspoon ginger

· 1/2 cup quick-cooking oats

· 2 tablespoons gluten

· 2 teaspoons celery seeds

· 1 package active dry yeast

Direction:

1.Add all ingredients to the machine pan.

2.Select basic bread setting.

Nutrition:

· Calories: 73

· Total fat: 3.6 g (0 g sat. fat)

· Carbohydrates: 8 g

· Fiber: 0

· Protein: 2.6 g

Orange Cappuccino Bread

Preparation time: 10 minutes

Cooking time: 3 hours

Servings: 1 loaf

Ingredients:

· 1 cup water

· 1 tablespoon instant coffee granules

· 2 tablespoons butter or margarine, softened

· 1 teaspoon grated orange peel

· 3 cups Bread flour

· 2 tablespoons dry milk

· 1/4 cup sugar

· 1 ¼ teaspoon salt

· 2 ¼ teaspoons bread machine or quick active dry yeast

Direction:

1.Add all ingredients to the machine pan.

2.Select Basic bread setting.

Nutrition:

· Calories:155

· Total fat: 2 g (1 g sat. fat)

· Carbohydrates: 31g

· Fiber: 1 g

· Protein: 4 g

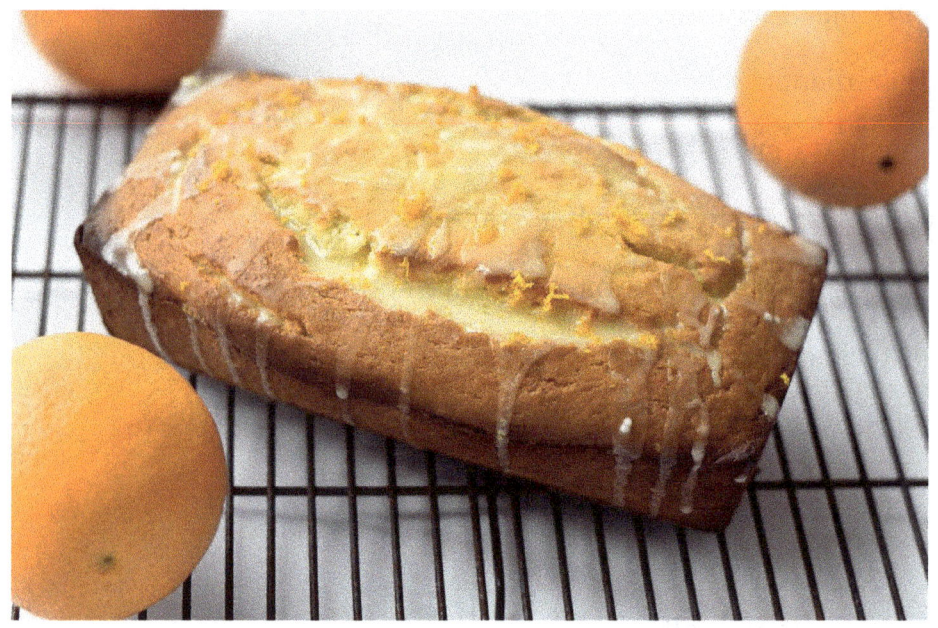

Red Hot Cinnamon Bread

Preparation time: 5 minutes

Cooking time: 3 hours

Servings: 1 loaf

Ingredients:

· 1/4 cup lukewarm water

· 1/2 cup lukewarm milk

· 1/4 cup softened butter

· 2 ¼ teaspoons instant yeast

· 1 ¼ teaspoons salt

· 1/4 cup sugar

· 1 teaspoon vanilla

· 1 large egg, lightly beaten

· 3 cups all-purpose flour

· 1/2 cup Cinnamon Red Hot candies

Direction:

1.Add ingredients to bread machine pan except for candy.

2.Choose Dough setting.

3.After the cycle is over, turn the dough out into a bowl and cover, let it rise for 45 minutes to one hour.

4.Gently punch down dough and shape it into a rectangle.

5.Knead in the cinnamon candies 1/3 at a time.

6.Shape the dough into a loaf and place in a greased or parchment-lined loaf pan.

7.Line the pan loosely with lightly greased plastic wrap, and allow a second rise for 40-50 minutes.

8.Preheat oven to 350°F.

9.Bake 30-40 minutes.

10. Remove and cool on a wire rack before slicing.

Nutrition:

· Calories: 207

· Total fat: 6.9 g (4.1 g sat. fat)

· Carbohydrates: 30 g.

· Fiber: 1 g

· Protein: 4.6 g

Cottage Cheese Bread

Preparation time: 10 minutes

Cooking time: 3 hours

Servings: 1 loaf

Ingredients:

· 1/2 cup water

· 1 cup cottage cheese

· 2 tablespoons margarine

· 1 egg

· 1 tablespoon white sugar

· 1/4 teaspoon baking soda

· 1 teaspoon salt

· 3 cups bread flour

· 2 ½ teaspoons active dry yeast

Direction:

1.Add all ingredients to the machine pan. Follow the order suggested by the manufacturer.

2.Select Basic bread setting.

Tip: If the dough is too sticky, add up to ½ cup more flour.

Nutrition:

· Calories: 171

· Total fat: 3.6 g (1 g sat. fat)

· Carb: 26 g

· Fiber: 1 g

· Protein: 7.3 g

Easy Bread for keto diet

Preparation time: 9 minutes

Cooking time: 21 min

Servings: 5

Ingredients:

· 6 large eggs

· 2/3 cup almond flour or almond supper

· 1/3 cup coconut flour

· 3 teaspoon coconut oil

· 1/2 cup unsalted margarine

· 2 teaspoons heating powder

· 1 teaspoon salt margarine or an olive oil shower

Directions:

1.Crack 6 large eggs into a food processor or blending bowl and mix well. Then add the almond flour or almond supper and the coconut flour.

2.Melt the coconut oil and margarine in the microwave and add them to the blend. Then add the salt and heating powder and blend or mix everything completely. Let it aside for 10-15 minutes so the blend thickens while you preheat your broiler to 350° F.

3.Coat a 9" x 5" heating tin with margarine or an olive oil shower and add your thickened blend to the tin. Pop the tin into the broiler and heat for 40 minutes. Haul the bread out when it turns a brilliant dark colored on top and let it cool on a rack.

Nutrition:

· Calories: 220

· Carbohydrates: 4 g

· Net Carbohydrates: 2.5 g

· Fiber: 4 g

· Fat: 12 g

· Protein: 8 g

Sauerkraut Rye Bread

Preparation time: 5 minutes

Cooking time: 3 hours

Servings: 1 loaf

Ingredients:

· 1 cup sauerkraut – rinsed and drained

· 3/4 cup warm water

· 1 ½ tablespoons molasses

· 1 ½ tablespoons butter

· 1 ½ tablespoons brown sugar

· 1 teaspoon caraway seed

· 1 ½ teaspoons salt

· 1 cup rye flour

· 2 cups bread flour

· 1 ½ teaspoons active dry yeast

Direction:

1.Add all ingredients to the machine pan.

2.Select Basic bread setting.

Nutrition:

•Calories: 74

•Total fat: 1.8 g (0 g sat. fat),

•Carbs: 12 g

•Fiber: 1 g

•Protein: 1.8 g

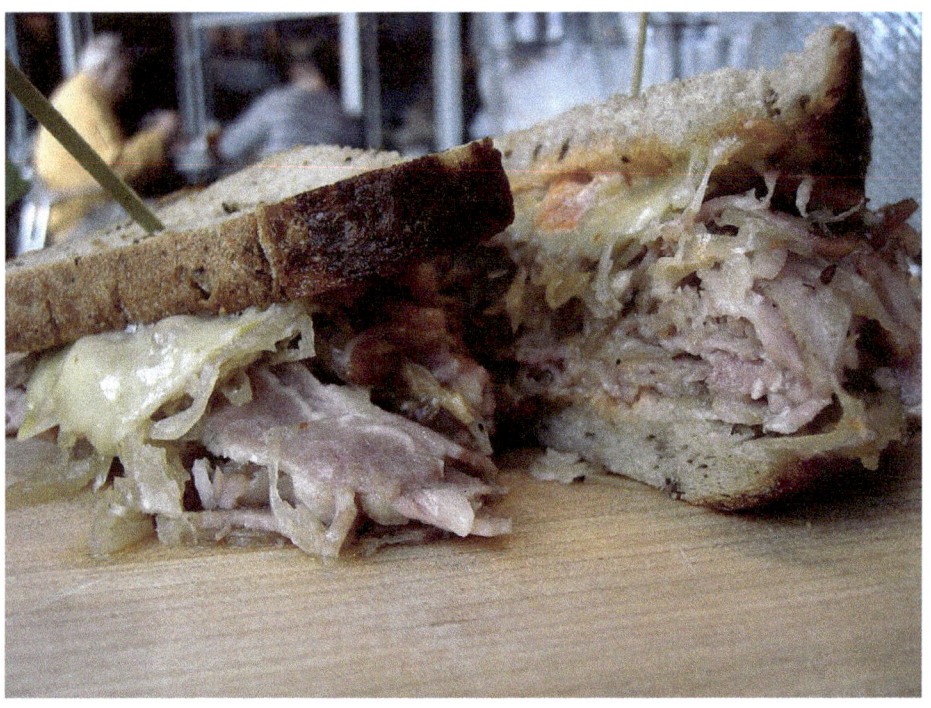

Keto Blueberry-Banana Loaf

Preparation time: 10 minutes

Cooking time: 2 hours 20 minutes

Total Time: 2 hours 30 minutes

Servings: 12 slices

Ingredients:

· ½ cup warm water

· 1 tablespoon almond milk, unsweetened

· 2 eggs, small

· 8 tablespoons Butter, melted, and unsalted

· 3 medium-sized mashed bananas

· 0.75 teaspoon stevia extract

· 2 cups almond flour

· ½ teaspoon salt

· 2 teaspoons Baking powder

· 1 teaspoon baking soda

· 1 cup frozen blueberries

Directions:

1.Prepare the ingredients. Beat the eggs and mash the bananas. Soften the butter in the microwave for 30 seconds. Mix the water and the milk.

2.Put the bananas, eggs, butter, water, and milk in the bread bucket.

3.Add in all dry ingredients except blueberries.

4.Start the bread machine by selecting Quick Bread, then close the lid. After the first kneading, open the lid and add in the blueberries. Close the lid and let the cycle continue until the end.

5.Once cooked, remove the bread from the bucket and let it cool in a cooling rack before slicing.

6.Serve.

Nutrition:

· Calories: 119

· Calories from fat: 90

· Total Fat: 9 g

· Total Carbohydrates: 9 g

· Net Carbohydrates: 7 g

· Protein: 2 g

Anise Almond Bread

Preparation time: 10 minutes

Cooking time: 3 hours

Servings: 1 loaf

Ingredients:

· 3/4 cup water

· 1 or 1/4 cup egg substitute

· 1/4 cup butter or margarine, softened

· 1/4 cup sugar

· 1/2 teaspoon salt

· 3 cups bread flour

· 1 teaspoon anise seed

· 2 teaspoons active dry yeast

· 1/2 cup almonds, chopped small

Direction:

1.Add all ingredients to the machine pan except almonds.

2.Select Basic bread setting.

3.After prompt, add almonds.

Nutrition:

· Calories:78

· Total fats: 4 g (1 g sat. fat)

· Carbohydrates: 7 g

· Fiber: 0

· Protein: 3 g

Three Ingredient Buttermilk Cornbread

Preparation time: 10 Minutes

Cooking time: 20 Minutes

Servings : 8

Ingredients:

· Vegetable oil as needed

· 1 1/2 cups buttermilk

· 1 1/2 cups cornmeal

· 1/2 cup all-purpose flour

Direction:

1.Preheat oven to 450 °F (230 °C). Pour enough oil into a skillet to coat the bottom; place into the oven.

2.Mix buttermilk, cornmeal, and flour together in a bowl until smooth. Remove skillet from oven; pour in buttermilk mixture.

3.Bake in the preheated oven until cornbread is golden brown— 20 to 25 minutes.

Nutrition:

· Calories: 157

The Best Corn Bread You'll Ever Eat

Preparation time: 5 Minutes

Cooking time: 30 Minutes

Servings: 8

Ingredients:

· 1 egg

· 1 1/3 cups milk

· 1/4 cup vegetable oil

· 2 cups self-rising corn meal mix

· 1 (8 ounces) can cream-style corn

· 1 cup sour cream

Direction:

1.Heat oven to 425 °F (220 °C). Grease a 9-inch iron skillet.

2.In a large bowl, beat the egg. Add milk, oil, sour cream, cream corn, and cornmeal mix; stir until cornmeal is just dampened. Pour batter into greased skillet.

3.Bake for 25 to 30 minutes, or until the knife inserted in the center comes out clean.

Nutrition:

· Calories: 328

· Total Fat: 15.9 g

· Total Carbohydrates: 40.8 g

· Protein: 6.4 g

Cauliflower Bread

Preparation time: 10 minutes

Cooking time: 54 minutes

Servings: 8

Ingredients:

· 3 cups cauliflower rice

· 10 large eggs

· 1/4 teaspoon cream of tartar

· 1 1/4 cups coconut flour

· 1 1/2 tablespoons gluten-free baking powder

· 1 teaspoon sea salt

· 6 tablespoons butter

· 6 cloves garlic (minced)

· 1 tablespoon fresh rosemary (chopped)

· 1 tablespoon fresh parsley (chopped)

Direction:

1.Start by preheating the oven to 350 °F and layer a loaf pan with parchment paper.

2.Place the cauliflower rice in a large bowl and cover it with a plastic sheet.

3.Cook the rice in the microwave for 4 minutes.

4.During this time, beat egg whites with cream of tartar in a bowl until it forms peaks.

5.Whisk coconut flour with egg yolks, salt, baking powder, garlic, and melted butter in a separate bowl.

6.Beat ¼ egg whites and blend the mixture in a food processor until incorporated.

7.Place the cauliflower rice in a kitchen towel and squeeze to absorb moisture from the rice.

8.Add the cauliflower rice to the food processor and pulse until well mixed.

9.Add rosemary and parsley.

10. Spread the cauliflower batter in a baking pan lined with parchment paper.

11. Bake the batter for 50 minutes until golden brown.

12. Slice and serve fresh.

Nutrition:

· Calories: 282

· Total Fat: 25.1 g

· Saturated Fat: 8.8 g

Garlic Focaccia Bread

Preparation time: 10 minutes

Cooking time: 20 minutes

Servings: 4

Ingredients:

Dry Ingredients:

· 1 cup almond flour

· ¼ cup coconut flour

· ½ teaspoon xanthan gum

· 1 teaspoon garlic powder

· 1 teaspoon flaky salt

· ½ teaspoon baking soda

· ½ teaspoon baking powder

Wet Ingredients:

•2 eggs

•1 tablespoon lemon juice

•2 teaspoons olive oil + 2 tablespoon olive oil to drizzle

Directions:

1.Start by preheating the oven to 350 °F.

2.Layer a baking sheet with parchment paper.

3.Now, whisk all the dry ingredients in a bowl.

4.Beat lemon juice, oil, and egg in a bowl until well incorporated.

5.Whisk in dry ingredients and mix well until it forms a dough.

6.Spread the dough on a baking sheet and cover it with aluminum foil.

7.Bake for 10 minutes approximately then remove the foil.

8.Drizzle olive oil on top and bake for another 10 minutes uncovered.

9.Garnish with basil and Italian seasoning.

10. Serve.

Nutrition:

· Calories: 301

· Total Fat: 26.3 g

· Saturated Fat: 14.8 g

· Total Carbohydrates: 2.6 g

· Fiber: 0.6 g

· Protein: 12 g

Macadamia Nut Bread

Preparation time: 10 minutes

Cooking time: 40 minutes

Servings: 6

Ingredients:

· 5 oz. macadamia nuts

· 5 large eggs

· ¼ cup coconut flour

· ½ teaspoon baking soda

· ½ teaspoon apple cider vinegar

Directions:

1.Start by preheating the oven to 350 °F.

2.Blend macadamia nuts in a food processor until it forms a nut butter.

3.Continue blending while adding eggs one by one until well incorporated.

4.Stir in apple cider vinegar, baking soda, and coconut flour.

5.Blend until well mixed and incorporated.

6.Grease a bread pan with cooking spray and spread the batter in a pan.

7.Bake the batter for 40 minutes approximately until golden brown.

8.Slice and serve.

Nutrition:

· Calories: 248

· Total Fat: 19.3 g

· Saturated Fat :4.8 g

· Total Carbs: 3.1 g

· Fibe:r 0.6 g

• Protein: 7.9 g

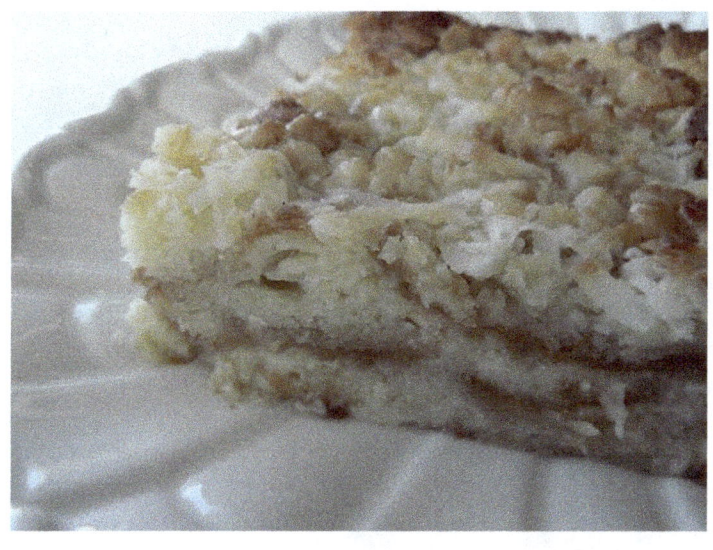

Sweet Challah Bread

Preparation time: 30 minutes

Cooking time: 45 minutes

Servings: 20

Ingredients:

· 1/4 cup dried berries

· 4 eggs

· 1 cup unflavored protein

· 1/2 of lemon zest

· 1/3 cup sukrin plus

· 1 teaspoon Xanthan

· 1.5 cup cream cheese

· 2 1/2 teaspoons baking powder

· 4 tablespoons butter

· 1/3 teaspoon baking soda

· 4 tablespoons heavy cream

· 1/2 teaspoon salt

· 4 tablespoons oil

· 2/3 cup vanilla protein

Directions:

1.Add all ingredients to the Bread Machine.

2.Select Dough setting and press Start. Mix the ingredients for about 4-5 minutes. After that press the stop button.

3.Smooth out the top of the loaf. Choose Bake mode and press Start. Let it bake for about 40 minutes.

4.Remove bread from the bread machine and let it rest for 10 minutes. Enjoy!

Nutrition:

· Calories:158

· Fat: 13 g

· Total carbohydrates: 2 g

· Protein: 9 g